Trust Me, I'm a Diet

Unhealthy. Unrealistic. Unsustainable.

Michael Vincent

Table of Contents

Introduction

Why do people diet?

Because they love rice cakes?

Because they just can't wait to get into their bran cereal the next morning? (Ha!)

Chances are good that it's not the above. In fact, the odds are rather high that nobody even likes dieting.

We diet because we want to look good, and enjoy the health benefits that come along with being our optimal shape. Those health benefits include reducing the risks of heart disease, diabetes and other conditions that are exacerbated by carrying unnecessary weight.

The reality is that there is such a huge demand to lose weight all over the world that it has become a billion-dollar industry. No matter where you live, if you walk into a store, you are bound to see products clearly marked sugar-free or fat-free for weight-loss.

If you go online, weight-loss ads will pop up without provocation. If you visit a bookstore, there is an entire section dedicated to weight-loss and dieting!

With each new fad diet that gains popularity, it becomes increasingly difficult to know which one to follow. Many diets directly contradict one another, each having their own claimed "success stories." With that said, they also each carry their own fair share of failures, most of which you will never find out about.

If each of these diets is so successful, why do so many people still struggle to lose weight? The reason is that almost every one of these diets is unsustainable.

If you want to lose weight (not only to look fashionable on your Facebook page by telling everyone that you're part of the latest fad), I mean really want to lose weight, the way to do it is actually very simple.

Are you ready?

The best way to drop some pounds is through correct diet and correct exercise.

If you read that carefully, the phrase used was correct diet – not diet. This means the overall way that you eat, as well as your lifestyle, need to improve.

Jumping from one fad diet to the next is the worst possible thing you can do for your health (not to mention your weight). What you need is a permanent lifestyle change that includes all the right foods with a perfect mix of activities that you enjoy.

Here's the background on it:

Nutrition is everything. It affects your mood, your body composition, and most importantly, your health. Proper nutrition not only nourishes the body, but also has a proven positive effect on your mental state.

The correct diet for your body will raise your energy levels, improve cardiovascular health and streamline digestion, as well as nourish your skin and boost overall quality of life.

Although a good diet will always trump exercise, putting them together is the most effective way to improve your body composition and health.

If this sounds like something that makes sense, keep reading. We're about to delve deep into the very idea of dieting, unpacking it one layer at a time. At the end of it all, you will be left with a better understanding of what it all does to your body, and the healthiest way for you to lose weight correctly.

<u>Chapter One</u> –

It's good to be a loser!

"What is so bad about all those popular diets? I hear they work for so many people."

In many cases, it is not the diet itself that is the problem. Quite often, the principles behind it are good and the advice is sound.

The problem is with the way that people follow them and how the advice is implemented.

The mental definition that most people have of the word "diet" is that it is a short-term thing. Once the diet is over and some weight has been lost, you get back to eating the way you always have. Right?

Therein lies your problem. Switching from one extreme to the other creates a terrible cycle of losing weight and then picking it up again, sometimes adding more weight than you actually lost. This is known as the yoyo effect or yoyo dieting, and has severe health implications.

Each time you change the way that you eat, your body is forced to change the way that it metabolizes food. Different foods in different quantities are digested differently. Interestingly, even the temperature of the food affects the composition and, in turn, the way that it is digested by your body.

In some cases, certain diets entirely change the type of food that your body burns for energy. This can be very useful; however, it needs to be followed strictly and for an extended period of time (usually indefinitely, in order for results to be sustained).

As the demands of a busy lifestyle force us to skip meals or grab unhealthy options as a last resort, all the positive effects of the diet are not only halted, but reversed.

Think of it this way: your body doesn't know that you are on a diet. As far as your brain is concerned, if you are eating less, it is because there is a shortage of food. This means that your metabolism slows down, making the most of any calories that you get in.

When your diet is over (or you give up due to not seeing results quickly enough), your body stockpiles all the excess calories and turns them into fat for storage. This is because you have taught it that there might be another shortage of food in the future, and it needs to prepare. Your brain's function is solely to keep you alive in the short term, with these efforts often being counter-productive in the long term.

Diets work differently for different people, even if they are followed exactly the same way. They are often affected by age, culture, the types and quality of food offered in different areas, as well as medication and personal preference.

What's interesting is that studies have shown that if you take two people from different countries and place them together, giving them exactly the same food for the same amount of time without any external influences such as medication, the diet will still have a different effect on them. The possible reasons for this include body composition and years of previous conditioning that have caused digestion to function a certain way.

What can we take from this?

The results of a diet cannot be guaranteed, as they affect every person in a unique way. You may even find that you actually gain weight from a diet that your friend has lost much weight on! It's not an exact science.

Furthermore, diets are not sustainable or healthy on a physical or a mental level. Drastically reducing the amount of food that your body takes in has been found to put your body in a state of anxiety. In this event, excess cortisol is produced, and chronic psychological stress usually accompanies it. These two results combined have an excessive effect not on weight loss, but weight gain. It has been clinically proven that sudden and excessive dieting is counter-productive!

The psychological effect that a diet has on your body may last much longer than the diet itself. Diets have been known to cause eating disorders, over eating or under eating. Chronic undereating becomes a diagnosable condition such as anorexia or bulimia nervosa. In extreme cases, the patients suffering from these diseases starve themselves to the point where their body shuts down and they die.

Chronic over-eating is one of the leading causes of obesity, a state which has been linked to a number of conditions such as diabetes, heart attacks and strokes, as well as high blood pressure. If not managed correctly, any one of these conditions can be fatal, due to the excessive strain that the excess weight places on the body.

When the body runs out of places to store fat, it builds up around the heart and other organs, as well as in the arteries. This makes it increasingly difficult for the body to perform at optimal levels. The state of stress causes extra cortisol to be produced, which, in turn, leads to additional weight gain. It becomes a vicious cycle that often spirals out of control.

In light of this, what do we do?

As it has been proven time and again that one diet does not work for everyone, diets should be avoided as a rule of thumb. In many cases, they cause more harm than good!

The way to lose weight is through eating in the manner that is correct for your body type.

You need to ensure that the calories you are consuming are less than the calories your body needs to maintain all of the cells within it. By doing so, you force the body to start using some of the energy that has been stored as fat – which is essentially why the fat was stored in the first place.

Consuming exactly the calories you need will maintain your weight, while consuming more than what your body needs will cause you to gain additional weight.

How to find out how many calories your body needs

It is surprisingly simple to work out exactly how many calories that your body needs in order to maintain its current shape. That being said, you do need to take into consideration any exercise that you are doing, as this burns additional calories.

Step One

Start by getting an accurate reading of your weight. Ensure that you have it in pounds, by converting from kilograms or stone if necessary. Multiply this amount by 11. This is the number of calories that your body needs per day in order to sustain all its cells.

Step Two

Unless you spend all day in bed, this amount needs to be adjusted to account for normal daily activities. Multiply the calories you calculated in step one by 1.5.

If you do no physical activity other than the normal daily tasks, you are done. This is the daily number of calories that your body needs to sustain itself.

Step Three

If you lift weights, multiply the number of minutes per week you spend lifting weights by 5. For example, if you lift weights three times a week for 30 minutes per session, you would need to calculate 90 (minutes) multiplied by 5.

Step Four

If you run, cycle or do any other high intensity exercise, this needs to be considered as well. Multiply the number of minutes per week that you any of these activities by 8.

Step Five

Add the values that you worked out in step three and four together. Then, divide this amount by 7 to get your daily average.

Step Six

Take the number of calories you calculated in step two, and add this to the figure you just worked out in step five. Together, this will provide you with a pretty accurate number of calories that your body needs each day just to sustain itself.

How much less should I be eating in order to lose weight?

If you are looking to lose weight, it is important not to eat too much, but also not to eat too little.

If you know how much weight you can safely lose per week, you can calculate exactly how much less calories you need to be eating. It is almost an exact science. If you are not sure how much you can safely lose per week, consult with your physician. A general rule of thumb is that you should not lose more than 1% of your total body weight per week.

Once you know how much you can drop per week without negatively affecting your health, here is how you work out what that means in calories.

One pound of fat is equal to 3500 calories. If you need to lose two pounds per week, that would mean you need to eat 7000 less calories per week. 7000 calories divided by 7 days in a week gives you 1000 less calories per day.

In other words, the number of calories you need to subtract from your daily calorie requirements is:

[Pounds to lose per week X 3500] divided by 7.

Isn't it difficult and time consuming to count calories?

Yes, counting calories can take up additional time, but it isn't as difficult as you may think. The best way to manage your calorie intake is simply to plan your meals ahead of time.

Once you know how many calories are in your favorite sandwich that you make all the time, it becomes easy to do a quick mental calculation on your calories for the day. You may find that it helps you to keep track by writing down what you eat, together with the corresponding calories. It can be a bit of a mental shift at first, but once you get into it, you won't be able to imagine life any other way.

Don't forget to include exercise

In order to get the best results, you need to change your lifestyle holistically. If you were not exercising previously, you need to make an effort to move more. As little as 30 minutes a day of moderate to high intensity exercise can have a profound effect on your weight loss. It also improves your body shape and builds muscle mass. This will lead to less stretch marks or excess skin being left over when the weight is gone.

Short summary of this chapter

It's good to be a loser, but you've got to lose weight in the correct way!

There is significant scientific research to support the idea that short term diets do more harm than good. Constant yoyo dieting can lead to mental and physical health issues that last substantially longer than the diet itself.

The best way to lose weight is to be aware of what you are eating. Ensure that the calories you consume are less than what your body needs to sustain itself. This forces your body to start using all the energy that it has been storing as fat.

It is important to know how many calories you need in a day and how much weight you can afford to lose safely. If you are not sure, consult with your physician before taking any drastic measures of you own.

Once you get into the right mindset, it becomes easier and can even be liberating. You will find that you lose weight without negatively affecting your quality of life or feeling as though you have been punished.

The most important factor in any weight loss journey is always to look at the long term. Would you pay $10 to get $5 back? Of course not! But you would jump at paying $5 to get $10 back.

The same concept applies to weight loss. It's got to be done gradually and over a long period of time, while incorporating exercise and healthy habits over the long term. Not only will you look and feel better, but you will be happier and enjoy a greater quality of life.

(Men's Fitness, 2017)

(Mayo Clinic, 2015)

<u>Chapter Two</u> –

What's out there?

Before you alter the way that you eat, a good starting point is always to do a little research on what is out there. Never start a diet without doing extensive reading up on what the experts say about it, and consulting with your doctor if you suffer from any health problems.

Ignore diets that suggest an absurd way of eating for a short period of time. Things to look out for are headlines that guarantee you will lose X number of kilos/pounds in X number of days/weeks. There are also a number of adverts for diets based around only one or very few food items, such as cabbage or eggs. Despite their attractive propositions, rather steer clear.

The correct diet for you will be balanced, included a variety of foods from different food groups. As there are differing theories, some may suggest more of a food group than another. Based on your specific health and body composition, not all of these diets will work for you. If you are not sure, rather see a dietician than take advice from just anyone.

In this chapter, you will find an outline of some of the most popular diets that are followed all over the world. Some of them have more scientific merit than others, offering varying levels of success for different people.

Each section will include a full description of the diet in question as well as a typical meal. From this information, you should find yourself in a better position to select which one, if any, would be the best for you. The ideal diet would fit naturally into your lifestyle and agree with any medical conditions that you may have.

The Atkins Diet

The founder of the Atkins diet is Robert Atkins, who is now deceased. His first book, Dr. Atkins' Vita-Nutrient Solution:

Nature's Answer to Drugs, was published in 1999. The Atkins diet was inspired by a paper Dr. Atkins read entitled Weight Reduction, written by Alfred W. Pennington in 1958. The paper was published in the Journal of the American Medical Association.

The principle behind the Atkins diet is high protein intake, high fat intake and low intake of carbohydrates. Although this may work for some people, there are also many people who report negative side effects of following this method of eating.

The Atkins diet is classified by many as a fad diet, as the scientific evidence behind its effectiveness is limited. Some research has found that the diet causes more weight gain than weight loss, possibly also being linked to heart disease.

A typical meal on the Atkins diet would include a seven-ounce pork chop with the bone in, half a cup of cauliflower florets, one cup of mixed greens and half a Hass avocado, all served with a sherry vinaigrette.

(Atkins.com, 2017)

(Wikipedia, 2017)

The Ketogenic Diet

The Ketogenic diet is comprised of eating high amounts fat, moderate or adequate amounts of protein, and low amounts of carbohydrates.

Interestingly, this diet is commonly prescribed as a treatment for epilepsy, recorded usage dating as far back as 400 BC.

By cutting out carbohydrates as much as possible and replacing them with fat, the body is forced to metabolize food differently. It starts to burn fat instead of carbohydrates for energy, which makes it significantly easier to lose weight. The name ketogenic means breaking down of fats for energy.

Many studies suggest that this is the way we were meant to digest food, dating back to the diet of the most primitive homo sapiens millions of years ago. Although this is quite commonly believed, there still isn't definitive evidence that proves this as being true.

A typical meal on this diet would include a chicken breast on salad greens, a dressing of oil and vinegar and a celery stalk for extra crunch.

(Dr. Andreas Eenfeldt, 2017)

(Wikipedia.org, 2017)

The Paleo Diet

The Paleo diet (also referred to as the caveman diet, the stone-age diet or the Paleolithic diet) is based on one very simple principle: Anything consumed as part of the diet needs to have been available to our early ancestors who were alive during the Paleolithic era.

The presumption is that human beings today are anatomically identical to homo sapiens that existed millions of years ago. As a result, in order to have the same athletic physique and optimal health, the diet recommends eating along the same lines that they did.

This would include fish, meat, eggs, fresh vegetables, nuts and seeds, and seasonal fruits in moderation. Any foods consumed need to be kept in their original form as much as possible – for example, using fresh tomatoes instead of canned tomatoes in sauces. Additives and preservatives are also to be avoided. Grains or any processed foods are to be avoided.

The Paleo diet is combined in most cases with an active lifestyle that contains low to moderate intensity exercise in favor of high-intensity exercise.

There is some debate on the scientific merit of this diet, as it is difficult to prove wither modern-day human beings have the same digestive systems as prehistoric human beings. Some evidence argues for it, while other evidence argues against it.

On a whole, the Paleo diet has had far greater success in terms of people benefited than other diets considered to be fads.

A typical Paleo breakfast would include two fried eggs, a handful of unsalted nuts or seeds, a handful of berries and some fresh vegetables. Supporters of the diet are in two camps about whether to include dairy or not, although those that exclude dairy commonly suffer from a calcium deficiency.

(Kamb, 2010)

(Wikipedia.org, 2017)

The Vegetarian Diet

There are numerous subsets of the vegetarian diet, having split in different directions over time. As a general rule, 50 percent of the diet would be made up carbohydrates, with fats and protein making up the remaining 50 percent.

The most common form of the vegetarian diet is lacto-ovo-vegetarian. People who follow this eat both dairy products and eggs, but entirely avoid all types of meat.

Those that eat dairy products but avoid eggs and meat are termed lacto-vegetarians.

Others eat eggs but avoid dairy products and meat. These are referred to as ovo-vegetarians.

There is a fourth group, however many believe that it should not be considered vegetarian as it defies the definition of not eating meat. People who follow this diet are called pesco-pollo vegetarians, as they avoid red meat but eat chicken and fish.

For the stricter vegetarians, they need to supplement their diet with additional protein as they do not consume enough protein to meet their daily dietary requirements. In these cases, they often add additional sources of protein from quinoa, buckwheat and soy, as well as beans, certain forms of rice, and hummus.

Vegetarians enjoy a large variety of food options, as there are vegetarian alternatives to most meat products such as burgers or sausages.

A typical vegetarian meal would include rice, vegetables, beans and/or eggs, depending on the subtype.

(The Vegetarian Society, 2016)

The Vegan Diet

The vegan diet is very similar to the vegetarian diet, although it is significantly stricter.

Vegans do not consume any type of meat or meat products, eggs or dairy. They also avoid all products made from animal by-products, such as leather. In many cases, vegans also avoid gelatin as it is made from boiling hide, cartilage and bones of animals.

The vegan diet is high in carbohydrates, with varying levels of protein and fat. Vegans do not follow a strict outline when it comes to what amounts of different foods they eat. Instead, the diet is focused on the foods that they do not eat, with almost free reign on the rest.

(Health Line, 2017)

The Weight Watchers Diet

The Weight Watchers diet provides an interesting and refreshing change to the majority of diets that are out there.

The weight-loss system is entirely based off points, guiding you towards healthier food choices. Weight Watchers provides a strong support system, offering diet suggestions and promoting positive lifestyle change.

While enrolled with Weight Watchers, you meet with the rest of the group for a weekly weigh-in and a discussion about achieving your weight-loss goals. The support and encouragement of the other members often plays a huge part, directly impacting motivations levels and results.

Weight Watches embraces the concept that losing weight is as much a mental challenge as it is a physical one, providing all the help that is needed on both fronts.

Although you need to be near a Weight Watchers center in order to be a part of the program, they have branches and centers all over the world.

A typical Weight Watchers meal is carefully calorie-controlled. An example of this would be a tuna pasta salad with a specific amount of tuna, mayonnaise, salad greens and pasta.

(Weight Watchers UK, 2017)

Intermittent Fasting

Although not a diet in the usual sense, intermittent fasting can play a huge role in assisting with weight loss.

The concept behind intermittent fasting is eating one's meals in a shorter space of time, in order to consume fewer calories for the day. This window is typically eight hours long, yet it can be changed based on your schedule and preferences.

Interestingly, intermittent fasting has a profound positive mental effect as well. Few people realize the amount of energy and resources that it takes for the body to digest food. A much more complex procedure than we give credit for, this highly-taxing activity makes it difficult for the body to do anything else at the same time.

This is often the reason why we feel sluggish and struggle to focus after a large meal. This effect is also greatly amplified by the type of foods we eat. For example, a salad will have less of this effect, whereas a starchy meal will drain an enormous amount of energy.

Intermittent fasting allows the body to get the digestion out of the way, freeing up resources for other mental or physical activity. This streamlines the body's processes, allowing it to focus on one thing at a time.

Many people experience a profound boost in their mental ability during intermittent fasting, often reporting a feeling on enhanced mental state and clearer thinking ability. It does not require a large change in lifestyle, and thus can work for many people.

(Clear, 2017)

The bottom line on all of the above diets

All of these diets have success stories, and have worked for many people all around the world. In the same token, all of them have just as many failures, and those are the ones you conveniently never learn of.

What is the diet that works? The only diet that will ever work for you is the lifestyle that is sustainable. You cannot claim a diet is effective if you immediately gain weight thereafter. You are not just back where you started, you are in a worse-off position in that situation.

If you are looking to lose weight, you need to change your thinking about food and change your lifestyle. Create a diet for yourself that you will be able to follow for the rest of your life. This needs to be a diet that you enjoy, and that doesn't feel like a punishment. Combine exercise and activity into it, and you've got a winning blueprint for success.

Weight-loss buzz words and key lifestyle phrases

Before we move onto the next chapter, let's take a look at some of the buzz words that we have used so far. It is important that you fully understand all of these concepts in order to make the most of this book!

What is a calorie?

A calorie is a unit that is used to describe the amount of energy you will receive from a specific food source. Every food source has a different number of calories, and thus will provide you with a different amount of energy.

As a general rule, fat contains twice as many calories per gram than proteins or carbohydrates. This makes it an efficient way for the body to store energy, but also a quick way to gain weight if you eat it! The average gram of fat contains 9 calories, whereas the average gram of protein contains only 4 calories.

(NHS Choices, 2016)

What is a carbohydrate?

For the average person, carbohydrates are the quickest source of energy that we can consume. They come in two main forms, sugars and starches, yet are also made up of fibers found in grains, fruits and vegetables.

Many diets suggest greatly limiting the amount of carbohydrates that you eat. The main reasons for this is that people generally consume far more than necessary, and also the adverse health effects that many carbohydrates cause.

That being said, carbohydrates as a whole are not unhealthy – they actually form a vital part of the average person's diet.

(Szalay, 2017)

What is fat?

Fat is not the villain that people speak of it as. It is an essential requirement of every diet, as it is important for correct brain functioning as well as body insulation.

That being said, there are several different types of fat, some considered healthy and some undoubtedly unhealthy.

The simplest way to remember the difference is that healthy fats are generally unprocessed and found naturally. Examples of foods that include healthy fats are avocados, omega three and six fatty acids (mainly found in fish), whole eggs and nuts. Olive oil is also considered a healthy fat.

Animal fats are considered unhealthy when consumed in large amounts. Examples of these are fatty cuts of pork, lamb or beef, or poultry skin.

Processed foods commonly contain a scarily-high amount of unhealthy fats. In order to avoid seed oils and trans fats, it is best to avoid processed foods altogether.

(SkillsYouNeed.com, 2017)

What is protein?

Protein is a nutrient that is essential for building muscle mass, and usually makes up about 15% of our body mass. It is predominantly found in all types of meats, yet also occurs in dairy products, beans, eggs, certain plant seeds and nuts.

Many diets contain large amounts of protein as it contains less calories than fat and is less likely to be stored for energy. People that spend a lot of time exercising commonly need a greater amount of protein in order to provide support for their muscles.

In order to lose weight, it is recommended that the proteins consumed are lean, which means that they are not as high in saturated fats. A few examples of suitable proteins are chicken or lean beef with all excess fat trimmed off, and low-fat dairy products. Avoid processed meats such as sausages, salami or bacon.

(Slazay, 2015)

What is gluten free?

Gluten is a protein found in certain grains and grain-based products. It is present in wheat, barley and rye, as well as in triticale which is a cross between wheat and rye. Gluten often irritates the lining of the gut, and thus many diets recommend avoiding it. For people with gluten sensitivity, the immune system goes as far as to attack gluten proteins, causing a number of health problems such as bloating, headaches, fatigue and diarrhea.

Gluten-free foods are easier to digest and kinder on the gut. It has also been found that a diet free from gluten offers the benefits of increased energy and focus.

There are a number of starches that are a good substitute, such as rice, potatoes, corn and soy. An important thing to note is that people who struggle with gluten intolerance are often sensitive to lectin as well, which is present in rice, many fruits and vegetables, and beans, amongst other things.

(Gluten-Free Living, 2017)

<u>Chapter Three –</u>

Why Do Diets Fail?

For every diet that the average person goes on, instead of losing weight, they gain 11 pounds. Quite often, weight that is lost is comprised of muscle and fat, yet when the weight is regained, only the fat returns.

Due to the fact that muscle burns significantly more calories than fat (seven times more, to be precise), their metabolism is slower than it was when they started. This means that they need even less calories than before to maintain their weight, meaning that even if they eat much less than they used to, they still don't lose weight!

The reason why most diets fail is a general lack of knowledge in the inner workings of the body while putting it through these measures. If we all knew the damage that fad dieting caused to our bodies, far, far less of us would follow them. It would put millions of blogs, magazines, authors and companies out of business.

The key to effective weight loss is not by starving yourself, but by reducing your appetite naturally. The unbalanced and out-of-control hormones in your brain that drive hunger and overeating can be stabilized, and it is all through correct food choices, active decisions and lifestyle.

Secondly, metabolism needs to be sped up to burn more calories. This may not be easy, as it is the exact opposite of the results fad diets have on the human body. You will need to undo many years of following the incorrect advice.

The best way to be successful in your new healthy lifestyle diet is to understand why all the other ones fail. Below are the top reasons why.

1. You're not using science to control your appetite

Appetite should not be controlled by willpower. You cannot hold your breath forever, just like you cannot starve yourself forever. This method of dieting is simply not sustainable.

Embrace the fact that hunger is a science, caused by a chemical reaction in your brain. Hunger is triggered by eating less, which is unfortunately what most diets advise you to do.

By not eating, you are going against every instinct your body has, and everything that your very DNA is telling you to do. Because of this, your body will do anything it can to get you to eat, all the while trying to get as much energy as it possibly can from what you do eat.

What's more, contrary to what is advertised all over the world, certain foods such as low-fat, sugary or high-carb foods actually increase hunger, while at the same time slowing down your metabolism.

Here's what you do to combat this:

Ensure that you eat only enough to satisfy your appetite. Keep in mind that these need to be whole, fresh foods.

Consume protein for breakfast, and ensure that you don't eat anything in the three hours prior to going to bed.

Remember that your meals need to balance blood sugar and reduce insulin levels, so be careful to plan them accordingly.

The perfect meal outline is a combination of protein and healthy fats with non-starchy, low-glycemic carbohydrates such as vegetables and fruits. If desired, you can add a small amount of grains or beans, yet not more than half a cup cooked volume.

The reason why this meal is effective is primarily due to the fact that protein, fat and fiber slow insulin spikes.

2. You take calories on face value

Never forget that calories are not all equal. Some cause weight gain, and some cause weight loss. The most important thing to remember is that any foods that cause an insulin spike trigger a shift in your metabolism. Examples of these foods include sugar, flour, grains, fruit and beans. In turn, the insulin released then removes the sugary fuel from your blood and deposits it directly into your fat cells – usually the ones around your stomach!

With a bloodstream devoid of fuel, your brain signals a hunger response and you eat more – even though less than an hour ago you successfully tackled a lasagna or drank a large Coke.

Don't forget that two things happen when your body thinks you are starving: hunger is stepped up and metabolism is stepped down.

If you've ever wondered why you're hungry again less than an hour after eating, you've just learnt the reason.

Here's what you do to combat this:

Build the staples of your diet from low-glycemic foods – as low as you possibly can. Good examples are chicken, fish, seeds, nuts, grass-fed meats and low-glycemic veggies.

Avoid grains as much as possible, consuming less than half a cup a day.

Treat sugar as a drug and avoid it at all costs. Only consume very small doses and only when you absolutely cannot get around it.

Avoid artificial sweeteners as much as possible. Although they don't contain many carbohydrates (if any), they do have other negative effects on the body. These include triggering sweet receptors and hunger, as well as slowing your metabolism – which ultimately leads to type two diabetes and/or obesity.

3. You subscribe to the low-fat hype

Low-fat really isn't all it's cut out to be. In fact, a low-fat diet can have more of a negative effect than a positive one when it comes to diet and weight-loss.

Although many people still maintain that egg-yolks are to be avoided at all costs, and that a low-fat diet is the key to weight-loss, it simply isn't true.

Let's use America over the last 30 years as a case study. Although low-fat was widely prescribed as a good diet to follow for weight-loss, the population is more overweight than it ever has been. What are the facts? 70% of Americans are overweight. Half of the American population has pre-diabetes or type two diabetes.

In a study on low-fat diets conducted by Harvard's Walter Willet, it was found that fat is surprisingly not the culprit of weight gain – the true offender is sugar. Further to this, scientist David Jenkins compared a low-carb (26%) high-fat

(43%) vegan diet with a low-fat vegan diet. The results were that the low-carb, high-fat diet had greater success in weight-loss as well as the reduction of cardio-vascular risk factors, when compared to the vegan low-fat diet.

The high-fat study group lost four more pounds than the low-fat group, also dropping their cholesterol levels by an average of 10 points when following the high-fat diet.

Their respective research is supported by other studies, some proving that your metabolism can be increased by 300 calories a day by eating more fat and less carbs – still keeping the total number of calories consumed per day the same. Mark Hyman, MD, described this phenomenon as having the same effect as sitting on the couch and yet still getting the benefit of running each day for an hour.

Here's what you do to combat this:

Embrace the idea that fat is not your enemy. If anything, it is an ally. Fat boosts satiation while simultaneously speeding up your metabolism and assisting with weight-loss.

Include a serving of good fats with every meal.

Plan your meals to include vegetable fats. Examples of these include nuts, coconut butter, seeds, avocado, and coconut oil.

When eating animal fats, ensure that they are clean animal fats, such as chicken and grass-fed meats, egg yolks from organic eggs, and fish (wild salmon, herring, black cod, sardines) that contain omega 3 fats.

4. There is another reason and it requires medical help

If you are struggling to lose weight, it might not be your fault. There could be a reason independent of your diet or amount of exercise that is affecting your metabolism and weight-loss.

In most cases, the main culprit to weight gain or difficulty losing weight is a factor that causes inflammation. Inflammation commonly increases insulin resistance, which makes it difficult for extra weight to be lost.

Let's take a look at some of the leading causes of inflammation.

Quite often, inflammation is caused by food allergies or sensitivities that you weren't even aware you had. The most common of these are gluten and dairy intolerances. That being said, replacing regular cookies with gluten-free cookies will not solve the problem – cookies are still cookies and the unhealthy ingredients remain. If you suspect this is the case, cut out gluten or dairy from your already optimized lifestyle diet.

What else could it be?

You may have problems with your gut. Bad bugs in your intestine can cause various problems from inflammation to changing the way that your food is broken down and absorbed. These can be caused by excessive consumption of refined or high-sugar carbohydrates, a low-fiber diet or even from taking antibiotics or acid blockers.

Toxins can also be a significant cause. Common environmental chemicals can be "obesogens" – actively making you fatter. Examples of potential suspects are heavy metals, pesticides, pollution, household cleaners and even makeup. This theory is substantiated by a study where rats who were given a specific toxin gained weight – even though their food and exercise levels remained consistent.

Here's what you do to combat this:

Since it may be difficult for a doctor to pinpoint, do some work yourself in the hopes of discovering what the cause of weight gain may be.

Start by trying an elimination diet. Don't remove calories, but remove inflammatory foods from your diet. It is advisable to stat with the most common culprits, gluten and/or dairy, and ensure that you follow this strictly for a full three weeks. It is almost impossible to get accurate results in a shorter space of time.

Repair your gut by starving the bad bugs. Eat a low-glycemic, low-starch diet. Ensure that you take probiotics during this time to maintain the necessary bacteria that your body needs to digest food. If you are unsuccessful on your own, consider booking an appointment with a functional medicine doctor.

The third step is to detox your body and cleanse your life. A reduction of exposure to chemicals could have just the impact you are looking for.

Be sure to check your skin-care products for the chemicals that they contain, and switch to products that are hypoallergenic and as natural as possible. Failing that, look up recipes online to make your own toiletries. You make find them surprisingly helpful.

Use the Environmental Working Group as a reference point to help you reduce exposures to these chemicals, including in your food and household products. Ensure that your fish does not contain mercury. Add two cups of cruciferous vegetables such as broccoli to your daily meal planning. Failing all else, speak to a functional medicine doctor for assistance with your detox and weight loss program.

5. You didn't think it through and don't have a plan

In the majority of circumstances, good health is something that can be planned and followed through on. Health is not something that simply happens to you without your having any control over it.

Those that fail to plan for their own health naturally fail. Without a guideline and a set plan of action, how could you possibly achieve a goal? As with life in general, success is not automatic. You have to want it, and you have to work for it.

Here's what you do to combat this:

Once you have created a plan or "design" for how you wish to eat and live your life, it becomes a simple matter of following through on the promises that you made to yourself. There are many simple tools and tricks to make this easier, such as having the right ingredients in the house, or having a no-take-out policy. Find what works for you, and stick to it.

Create a travel food pack for when you know you're out for the day. This prevents you from getting hungry and purchasing the first food item sold by the nearest fast food outlet. Remember that your meal plan goes hand in hand with your exercise plan. Follow through on them together to achieve the best possible result. What's the use in doing something halfway?

Another proven method is finding someone to do it with. Be it your partner, a friend or even just an acquaintance that you share the common interest with, doing it together has been found to generate significantly better results. If you are unable to find someone in person, take a look at the many online support platforms for doing exactly what you are trying to do. Being part of a likeminded community can be a wholesome and rewarding experience.

Commit to designing your health every weekend for the upcoming week. This makes it much easier to follow through on, as you are already in the mindset of doing what you set out to do.

Once you have found a method that words for you, don't sit back and expect a miracle. You've got to plan for your health and you've got to work on it.

(Mark Hyman, 2016)

<u>Chapter Four –</u>

The Pill Problem

Let's kick this chapter off with a case study that almost all of us can relate to.

Meet Steven. A regular 28-year-old, Steven works an office job as a legal clerk for a relatively successful firm. His girlfriend has just told him that she is pregnant, and he is excited and nervous about this next stage of his life.

Knowing that he will soon have a family to provide for, Steven puts in extra hours and does all he can to get himself noticed at work. He knows there will be a promotion coming up in the next few months, and is doing all he can to get it.

With his girlfriend's family putting pressure on him to marry her, he knows he needs to put money aside for an engagement ring and upcoming wedding costs. As a combined result of the long hours, lack of sleep and increased stress levels, Steven hits burnout and falls ill.

The doctor prescribes some flu pills, and Steven takes the rest of the day off work, although booked off for three. The next day he's back at the office. He cannot afford to lose this promotion, and forces himself to work through the flu. The extra hours have him skipping meals; resorting to eating whatever is available at the office canteen.

As a result, Steven has picked up weight and is feeling sluggish, bloated and low on energy. This causes a direct drop in his performance levels, as well as making the occasional mistake at work. To his boss, Steven appears to be slacking off, and is not being seen in a good light.

Frustrated and short-tempered, Steven goes home and has an argument with his girlfriend about something trivial. He finds himself having a few drinks to calm himself down. Realizing that the added pressure has caused large levels of stress, Steven gets a prescription for ant-stress medication.

Whether Steven gets the promotion or not is no longer relevant. His physical and mental health have drastically declined based on a change in habits over only a short space of time.

Physicians today seldom do all-round checks nor offer holistic advice when it comes to our health. Instead, they prescribe pills from the hundreds of thousands that are currently available. Rather than providing lifestyle advice and recommendations to reduce stress levels, they hand out scripts to deal with it.

More and more people are on so many different types of medication that they struggle to keep track. The unfortunate truth is that, in many cases, the medication is not only unnecessary, but unhealthy as well.

Many pills have side effects worse than the conditions they are produced to treat! So why do we take them?

Humans have always loved the quick-fix solution; the fastest method with the least possible work required. Taking pills is substantially easier than taking a few steps back and trying to analyze where it all went wrong. Pills require no effort and no lifestyle change on our end. They are the easy way out and often nothing more than a band-aid fix to a much larger issue.

What about diet?

A diet based on bought bulk-made foods is the worst thing you can do to your body. There is no way for you to be sure of the quality or the freshness of the ingredients used. Combined with this, a lack of sleep and a stressful lifestyle is a recipe for disaster! Nevertheless, it is how most of us live our lives.

As a general statement, food prepared at home is better than anything you could buy. Anything mass-produced would generally contain additives and preservatives that you would not usually add in your own kitchen.

What's more, the quality of purchased food when it comes to nourishing your body falls embarrassingly far below the standards. Food served even in most hospitals contains limited nutritional value for our bodies.

Our digestive system is forced to sift through this gunk and somehow extract all of our daily nutritional requirements from it. You're right, it's just not possible, not to mention the amounts of strain these bad habits cause.

For those that can afford it, weight-loss surgery is often seen as the best option. Yes, it's another quick-fix! We're incredibly lazy as a species.

All of these issues could have been prevented by simply giving your body the nutrition it needs. I am not referring to a multivitamin, which is little more than yet another pill we swallow each and every day.

Nutrition needs to come from diet. It needs to come from eating a good variety of foods made up with a sizeable amount of fresh fruits and vegetables.

Combing the ease of which anyone can get pills (to treat almost anything) together with the strong desire to lose weight has created a whole new problem. Pharmaceuticals saw the gap decades ago, and have been selling "miracle" weight loss pills and products to consumers for years.

Although those products may work for people who are already on a strict energy-controlled diet, for the average consumer, they are no more than a waste of money. The problem is commonly in the way that the products are marketed. Consumers expect to take the pills and almost immediately start seeing and feeling results, as shown in the advertisements.

The fact is that there is no miracle formula to make the weight slide right off. It takes hard work and commitment to make it happen. With correct diet and exercise comes the correct lifestyle. Although this may be aided by supplements, in many cases, it is better in terms of health not to use them at all.

<u>Chapter Five –</u>

What Can We Agree On?

The Ketogenic diet instructs us to cut out carbs. The vegetarian diet recommends that all carbs be eaten. Why can't we call just get along?

The facts are that each diet has a degree of merit, however the majority of them are greatly contradictory. Perhaps the best method of deciding how to eat is to take the common advice that they all share.

Below are the diet choices that all of these diets can agree on, across the board.

Water is king

Every diet you will ever read up about will tell you how important water is for health and weight loss.

Refined carbohydrates are bad!

Refined carbohydrates contain little to zero fiber. In the creation of refined carbs, the final product is often shockingly far away from the raw materials used.

Examples of refined carbohydrates include:

- Table Sugar

- Corn Syrup

- Maple Syrup

- Most breads

- Doughs

- Waffles/pancakes, etc.

(Winston, 2017)

Sleep is vital for good health

We all know the feeling of having to get through the next day after a sleepless night. The only think on your mind is your bed!

The benefits of sleep are far greater than making you feel good. It is a vital aspect of a healthy lifestyle, having many proven benefits for your mind, heart, weight and other things, too.

What does enough sleep do for you?

It boosts memory.

In a process called consolidation, your mind actually revises through recent skills and information you learnt. This plays a large part in helping you remember important facts and master new talents. No matter what it is that you are trying to learn, a good night's rest plays a large part in it.

Sleep may improve longevity.

Studies have shown that less than six hours of sleep correlates with more deaths. As sleep boosts overall bodily functions, a recurring lack of sleep puts unnecessary strain on your body.

It brings down inflammation.

Inflammation is associated with many serious conditions such as heart disease, arthritis, diabetes and strokes. A 2010 study found that people who sleep six hours or less have a higher level of C-reactive protein (an inflammatory protein) present in their blood. This shows that more sleep helps to alleviate symptoms of inflammation.

Sleep also gets those creative juices flowing.

For the creative types, sleep is vital in order to create a break-taking work of art. For the corporate types, this creativity may help with strategic focus planning and innovative thinking. This is because it has been found that your brain re-structures your memories in your sleep, making way for enhanced creativity.

It improves athletic performance.

Sleep prepares you for strenuous activity by allowing your muscles time to rebuild and repair. A study conducted by Stanford university found that college football players who slept 10 hours or more per night noted a marked improvement in their athletic performance. Similar results were found for swimmers and tennis players.

Sleep improves cognitive performance.

Children between the ages of 10 and 16 who experienced difficulty sleeping were found to perform worse academically than those who slept enough. It has also been found that snoring and sleep apnea correlates to increased difficulty with attention and learning.

Sleep makes it easier to focus.

Interestingly, a lack of sleep in children causes hyperactivity, as opposed to the sleepiness experienced by adults. A study published in a 2009 journal, Pediatrics, noted that seven- to eight-year-old children who slept less than eight hours per night were frequently impulsive, hyperactive and inattentive. This increases the chances of sub-average academic performance.

It helps you lose weight effectively.

The University of Chicago found that adequate sleep changes the way we lose weight. Although both groups lost the same average amount of weight, the sleep-deprived group lost mainly muscle mass, whereas the other group lost 56% fat.

It helps to lower stress levels.

Countless studies have shown that adequate sleep allows keeps stress levels manageable. High levels of stress are commonly correlated to poor cardiovascular health.

Sleep helps depression.

Those who have depression experience less feelings of anxiety after having a good night's rest. On the same token, a lack of sleep has also been found to contribute negatively to depression.

(Sparacino, 2013)

Saturated or Trans-fat? Neither, thank you!

As discussed in Chapter One, fat is an essential part of our diet. Hence, our decision is not whether or not to include fats in our diet, but rather to select the types of fats that we choose to consume.

Trans fat is predominantly found in hydrogenated oils. As the average person is not familiar with the term, hydrogenation is the process of adding hydrogen to a liquid in order to turn it into a solid.

Trans fats are not found anywhere in nature and are not ideal for you.

As a general rule, oil that is liquid at room temperature is from plants. Oils solid at room temperature are from animals and contain very low nutritional value.

(A Calorie Counter, 2017)

Soft drinks are not something anybody should be drinking

Soft drinks are a poisonous combination of sugar, additives and preservatives. Even the sugar free varieties, although a better choice than the original varieties, should be cut out completely. Water is the healthiest and most readily accessible beverage – why would you drink anything else?

Zero-Calorie Foods

What is a zero-calorie food?

It is not possible for a food item to contain zero calories and still garner nutritional value from it. However, your digestive system burns calories just by digesting food, and sometimes the energy spent is more than the energy gained.

To explain the concept in layman's terms, if a celery stalk is worth 5 calories and you burn 8 calories from eating it, this means that you are actually losing weight while eating. What a pleasure!

These zero-calorie foods have a tremendous positive impact on your health, as they are packed with vitamins and minerals. What's more, they are relatively inexpensive, and may even save you a trip or two to the doctor.

Try to purchase your fresh fruits and vegetables from farmers' markets as much as possible. Not only are they farm-fresh, but they are generally organically grown and free from chemicals. You may even be treated to a story about the year's current crops. How's that for interacting with your food?

Keep in mind that you cannot eat a whole wheelbarrow full of these foods and still expect to reap the zero-calorie benefit. It's all relative to how much you eat and how you prepare it.

What are some zero-calorie foods?

Fruits:

Apples, apricots, grapefruit, oranges, strawberries, tangerines, watermelon

Vegetables:

Carrots, celery, onions, red bell peppers, spinach and other leafy greens, tomatoes

Asparagus, broccoli, cauliflower, green beans, kelp, mushrooms, zucchini and summer squash

(Levin, 2017)

Optimal health is a lifestyle choice

Although eating well is a vital part of it, optimal health extends farther than nutrition alone.

In order to transform your body, remember that your mind is equally important and that the two tie into one another.

Exercise is as much a mental challenge as it is a physical one. That being said, it is not necessary to push yourself to the limits and go flat out every time you exercise. In order to lose weight and improve your general health and wellbeing, all you need to do is move more.

Park farther away and walk the extra distance. Take the stairs instead of the lift. Kick your day off with a 30-minute yoga session or jog. Even playing in the pool with your kids counts as mild exercise.

As long as you are moving, however slowly, your body is burning calories. Oxygen is pumping through your muscles, improving tone and sculpting a better body.

Your body needs exercise, and it has been proven to reward you for it. Aerobic exercises (such as cycling, swimming and running) in particular have been found to not only release, but also produce serotonin. The feel-good hormone, serotonin is what puts that smile on your face after a good workout.

<u>Chapter Six –</u>

What are the facts?

What do I need to know when it comes to dieting for weight loss?

By this point, it is clear that following an existing diet is not the most effective way to lose weight, especially if the diet in question is considered a fad by authoritative sources.

That being said, you do still want to lose weight, so what is the best way to go about it?

With all the differing opinions on the correct way to eat, it's easy to get swept up in all the confusion. To make life easier, forget the rest and focus only on the following simple principles. If you follow them closely, not only will you lose weight the correct way (fat loss not muscle loss), but you will also notice higher energy levels, increased ability to concentrate and overall mood upliftment. It's an empowering process.

How do I know which foods I can and should be eating?

It's not much of a debate, although the answer is broad. The winner is real food.

Real food is organically grown and freshly made by you, in your own kitchen. It does not include any ingredients that can be found in a can or any other preserved state. It is not processed and does not contain MSG or other flavor enhancers.

Furthermore, real food should be consumed in the state as close as possible to how it would be found naturally. To clarify, if you are eating fruit, opt for fresh fruit instead of dried fruit.

Why? In its natural form, you are far less likely to consume too much of it. Use dried mango as an example – many people can eat 500g of dried mango without thinking twice, but few people would consume the same amount of the fruit fresh – which is two to four mangoes, depending on size. The scary truth is that dried mango contains more sugar, calories and carbohydrates than fresh mango. If you absolutely have to eat dried fruits, avoid the candied kinds that have added sugar. Rather purchase it from health stores, or dry your fresh fruit yourself in an oven.

When it comes to meats, strictly avoid any forms of processed meats and eliminate them completely from your diet. If you need any motivation to do this, take a look online at how processed meats are made. You may well shudder at all the animal parts that you have been eating over the years.

If you are not sure what meat is processed, here's a quick guideline: Any meat that has been cured, salted, smoked, canned or dried is considered processed by most standards.

Below is a list of the most common forms of processed meats that you really should not be eating (at all, ever).

- bacon

- beef jerky

- canned meat

- corned beef

- deli/luncheon meats

- frankfurters

- ham

- hot dogs

- meat-based preparations and sauces

- salami

- sausages

Eat plenty of vegetables and seasonal fruits in moderation

Most people will tell you that you need to eat as much fruit and vegetables as you can, but on face value, that is not necessarily good advice.

Not all vegetables are created equal. Many are starchy, such as:

- Corn

- Lima beans

- Peas

- Potatoes

- Sweet potatoes

- Winter squash

These vegetables should be consumed in moderation, although never cut out completely unless for a specific dietary reason. If desired, these can make up the starch of a meal instead of rice, pasta or any other non-vegetable starch.

In the previous chapter, there were vegetables noted under the heading of zero-calorie foods. You have significantly greater freedom with regards to the amount of these that you can eat. As these are not considered starchy vegetables, it is acceptable and recommended to all them to meals that do or do not contain starch.

(BBC News, 2015)

(University of Illinois Extension, 2014)

A few words on exercise

Exercise is vital in order to maintain a healthy weight, as well as lower the risk of contracting certain diseases, illness and/or being diagnosed with otherwise preventable medical conditions. Not only does it help you to burn calories, but it actively boosts serotonin levels and leaves you feeling great.

This has a huge and highly beneficial impact on the rest of your lifestyle, helping you to perform better at work and enjoy a happier outlook. It is key to losing weight, and the new and improved well-toned body will leave you feeling like a million bucks.

If you are not used to exercise, start small and build from there. Commit to getting just 30 minutes of activity in every day of the week, and you will already start to see results. The activity does not have to be high-intensity – even taking a stroll to the nearest convenience store instead of driving will do. Take your dogs for a walk, or enjoy a relaxed swim with friends or family. No matter what you do, as long as you are moving, you are doing it right.

With time, you can build on your exercise habits and they will feel like less of a chore. As your fitness levels improve and the results appear, you will look forward to the daily gym session or other activity. A few well-placed compliments from friends and colleagues don't hurt either!

If you are unable to exercise due to medical issues or injury, find a low-intensity activity that you can do. Push yourself to do a little every day, even if the activity may seem miniscule to others. Remember, you are not competing against them. You are competing against yourself.

Bed-ridden people can try out activities such as yoga (limited to what they are able to do). Disabled people can dabble in swimming, even it if is simply splashing in the water. Mentally-handicapped people have found great joy and value in engaging with animals, especially working with animals and horse-back riding.

The bottom line is that there is something for everyone. There is never an excuse to do nothing at all, especially if you are committed to making some positive changes in your life.

The importance of hydration

Every diet in the world will stress the importance of hydration, each one recommending an average of at least two liters of water per day.

However, as with your daily calorie needs, the amount of water that your body requires is dependent on a number of factors, such as your weight and activity level. It can also be influenced by the weather and humidity where you live, as much water is lost through sweating during normal daily activities.

In order to get an accurate personal daily water requirement, follow the steps below.

Start by getting an accurate reading of your weight, and note it down in pounds. Do a conversion if your country-specific norm is anything other than pounds.

Multiply your weight in pounds by 67%, or 0.67. This will provide you with the amount of water in ounces that your body needs each day.

This amount needs to be adjusted for exercise or any activity that causes you to sweat. Add 12 ounces of water for every 30 minutes of exercise that you do on average each day.

(Shaw, 2017)

How to drink more water

As many of us need actual reminding to drink water, here are a few good habits that you can pick up to get you on the right track.

Drink 2 cups (or 500ml) of water before each meal. This assists with digestion, as well as helps you to consume less food during the meal, actively boosting your weight loss. If this habit is followed through three times a day, you have already downed 50oz or 1.5 liters of water. This should make it significantly easier to make up the balance of your water requirement during the day.

Drink a glass of water before you fall asleep at night, and one first thing in the morning when you wake up.

Buy a special water bottle and use it to keep track of how much water you drink in a day. The larger the water container, the better. For example, if you need to drink 130 ounces of water per day and your bottle holds 34 ounces, you know you need to drink three and a half bottles in order to reach your goal.

If you struggle to drink plain water, infuse it with fruit, vegetables or mint leaves. A different taste makes it go down easier, as well as adding some additional vitamins to your diet. Many grocery chains also offer water enhancers, and many of them have the added bonus of being calorie-free.

Others suggest mixing it up with carbonated variants to make it more pleasant to drink. Carbonated water and even calorie-free flavored water are good alternatives to plain water.

(Mccaffrey, 2012)

No matter who you are, you need to get enough sleep!

The positive benefits of sleep were explained at length in the previous chapter, as well as the disastrous effects that arise from a lack thereof. Ensure that you are getting more than enough sleep each night in order to function at your optimum level.

Nutrition can preemptively fight disease

Our bodies are amazing things. Given the right tools, they are able to fight off sickness and disease in many cases before we are even aware that we were falling ill.

The most important thing your body needs in order to perform at its best is proper nutrition. Ensure that you are getting plenty of vitamins and minerals in, and your body will thank you. Less visits to the doctor also mean less time off work and more things get done. Once you are in the habit of eating properly, it will be very difficult to imagine that it was ever any other way.

With the added plus of looking fabulous, eating according to your body's needs can be truly life-changing.

Smoking: Why do it?

If you are serious about becoming healthier, it is important to have a holistic approach. Just like we snigger at the person at McDonalds who orders a double burger and fries with a diet coke, it is ridiculously counter-productive to eat well and exercise often yet nurse your smoking habit. In the United States alone, governmental statistics have shown that an average of 480,000 people die each year due to health conditions caused by smoking. In addition to this, it is estimated that smokers live an average of 10 years less than non-smokers.

If your health is not enough of a deterrent (yikes!), consider the financial cost of the habit. If a person smokes 3 packs a week at an average of $5,50 per pack, it adds up to a staggering $858 per year. Imagine what you could do with an extra $850 around Christmas time. It might even be enough for a weekend away with your partner.

Alcohol and weight loss

When it comes to alcoholic beverages, it's not the alcohol alone that carries all the calories, but rather the mixers and the cocktails that they are accompanied by. A 1.5oz (44ml) shot of spirits or hard tack such as gin, whiskey, tequila, vodka or rum contains an average of 100 calories. A 5oz (150ml) serving of wine offers roughly the same amount.

As soon as we start adding mixers and creating alcoholic concoctions, it becomes increasingly difficult to keep track of the number of calories consumed.

The problem with alcohol, however, is not limited to the number of calories it contains. In almost all cases, it has a significant behavioral impact as well.

As the key to a healthy lifestyle is diet, exercise and sleep, alcohol tends to wreak havoc on this delicate balance. Just one or two drinks increases your total calorie consumption, almost entirely does away with your motivation to exercise, as well as messes with your sleep cycles.

Once again, it comes to the point where you may find yourself asking, "Why do it?" Alcohol and smoking (not to mention drugs and other forms of substance dependence) makes it increasingly difficult to follow a healthy lifestyle. If losing weight and getting healthy is important to you, it may be time to take a serious look at your current lifestyle choices and make some tough decisions.

<u>Chapter Seven –</u>

What Can I Do About It?

You can start today.

Be more active. Get in the habit of moving more, even if it is to the end of the driveway and back. The hardest part is getting started. Once you have done that, you can build on it and take it from there.

You've got to take some time to yourself to get real and get serious. Perhaps get a pen and paper, and admit to yourself what you consider to be your biggest flaws. It is only in facing your obstacles that you will be able to overcome them. Remember that this is as much a mental journey as it is a physical one. Once you understand and respect that, you are halfway there.

Allow yourself some time to feel every emotion that comes over you. Feel it, appreciate it and understand it. It is necessary to do the extra work, as this is not a diet that you will be following for the next few weeks. You are laying the foundations for a lifestyle that you will carry with you for as long as you hope to live.

Understand that small changes do lead to bigger changes. Nobody can change overnight! Set yourself reasonable goals in realistic time frames, and take them one step at a time.

Remember that the only one that has complete control over your life, your future, your happiness and your body is you. You have the power of now, and the ability to make some positive movements in some amazing directions.

Believe in yourself. You've got to be your own biggest fan, because there will be times where it feels as though there aren't any other people supporting you. Understand and embrace it. That is okay. Each person has their own journey, and you're only in control of your own.

Forget what the internet and the TV says about how you can or how you should look. They don't know you, and you don't know them. As far as they are concerned, you are just another client that may buy into their products and make them richer.

The most important thing is that you live long and prosper, feeling comfortable in your own skin while doing so. You are not doing this for anybody other than yourself, so you certainly shouldn't be allowing someone else to make the rules.

The scale can be your friend or your enemy, and it all depends on your mindset about it. Keep in mind that the average person will fluctuate over 5lbs a day, so don't weigh yourself any more often than you absolutely need to! Remember that it's not just about that number on the display. It's about how you look and how you feel. If you are feeling better about yourself, your choices and your lifestyle, you have already won first prize.

Pay attention to the details discussed in this book and you will be on the right path. It is designed as a handbook and a guide; a friend that will remind you of your journey when you stray off the path. Don't forget that we are all human! We all get lost from time to time. It is your efforts to return to the correct path that matters.

75

<u>Chapter Eight</u> –

Do I have to exercise?

Exercise doesn't have to be scary. It doesn't have to be daunting, and it doesn't have to be a chore. If you feel that way about it, you are probably doing it wrong!

If you are at a stage in your life where you are doing absolutely no exercise, the worst thing you can do to yourself is plunge into a stringent workout regimen. It's no good for your body and certainly no good for your mental state – and you may find yourself pulling out in a very short space of time.

What do people do when they give up? They immediately revert back to their old habits. They decide that working out just isn't for them. They accept their weight and their potential shortened lifespan.

If you have reached this point in this book, it is probably fair to assume that you are not planning on giving up before truly having started. You are motivated enough to commit to a lifestyle change that you will carry with you for the rest of your life, reaping the rewards as the years progress.

Why is exercise important?

There is no way around exercise, and that is because it is absolutely vital in order for your body to function optimally.

When you don't exercise, a negative chain reaction takes place that gradually makes it harder for you to exercise. You will notice that your muscles weaken and become flabby. Your lungs and heart do not function optimally, and your joints are stiff and at risk of injury.

The longer you go without exercise, the worse these symptoms become. When you do start to exercise, it is much harder than it would have been if your body were used to the constant state of movement.

In light of this, in many ways, inactivity can be as unhealthy as smoking!

Here's what exercise actually does for you:

Exercise aids in disease prevention

As the human body is designed for movement, it needs exercise to remain healthy and physically fit. A frequent level of exercise plays a significant role in preventing heart disease, high blood pressure, cancer and diabetes, amongst other diseases. Furthermore, it betters your appearance and actually delays the process of aging – helping maintain a youthful vigor.

Exercise improves your stamina

Naturally, energy is required to maintain levels of exercise. Continued and rhythmic physical motion is known as aerobic exercise, examples of which being cycling and walking. This is an excellent form of exercise as it trains your body to use energy more efficiently, which improves stamina. As aerobic exercise is done more often, the body is able to return breathing rate and heart rate to normal in a shorter space of time. This is due to your body adjusting to the exercise; the improvement of your conditioning level.

Exercise tones and strengthens

Weight- and other forms of resistance training are excellent for muscle development. It also strengthens bones and ligaments, increasing endurance. As your muscles become firmer, you may receive comments that your posture has improved. Resistance training also minimizes the risk of injury, due to the bone and ligament reinforcement.

Exercise improves your flexibility

Stretching is another form of exercise, and one of the most important. It allows for greater flexibility which further reduces the risk of injury. If injury occurs, the recovery rate is often significantly faster for patients who were in the habit of stretching frequently.

As stretching keeps your body limber, these exercises create masked improvements in your ability to twist, reach and bend. This also improves posture, balance and coordination.

Stretching is widely known to relieve stiff and tense muscles, especially on the back or neck area. This has been found to create a profoundly relaxing effect as excess stress and tension is released.

Exercise aids in weight loss

Ah, the reason many of us exercise in the first place! Exercise burns calories, which assists in weight control. They key factor is to burn off more calories than you consume, which will cause you to lose excess weight.

Exercise boosts quality of life

Once a regular exercise schedule is maintained, you will begin to feel the positive impact that it is having on your physical and mental state. Not only does it keep you feeling and looking younger (even as the years progress), but it also lifts moods, reduces stress and aids in proper sleep cycles. You can't overstate the benefits of a good night's rest.

Several studies have linked frequent exercise to reduced symptoms of depression. Although there are many views as to how exactly it works, the results cannot be argued. A common theory is that exercise blocks negative thoughts by providing a distraction from daily troubles.

Exercising can provide a great opportunity for social contact when done with friends. Workouts have been found to be significantly more effective when completed with a workout partner, partially due to mutual encouragement and motivation.

Furthermore, exercise positively changes levels of chemicals in your brain. It has been found to release serotonin and endorphins, and reduce stress hormones.

(Armand Tecco, 2017)

(Better Health Channel, 2017)

How to start exercising

Beginning an exercise regime is not as easy as getting up and starting to work out. Below are a few guidelines to help get you going.

Cardiovascular / Aerobic exercise

When it comes to cardio, beginners often bite off more than they can chew. The best piece of advice is to start off slower than you think you should, which will allow your body the necessary time to adjust. A safe, effective and realistic number is three days per week. Start off with no more than 30 minutes per session, and don't push yourself beyond the limit of what is comfortable. The aim at this point is to settle into the habit of exercising three times a week at a comfortable pace. Only if desired should the intensity be increased, at a later stage.

When it comes to beginner's cardio, walking is one of the best exercises. It can be done anywhere at any intensity, for any length of time. It is scientifically proven to be good for your body, offering a variety of benefits as previously detailed.

If you have experience in exercise and are just looking for a little more structure, a good rule of thumb to follow is to do aerobic (cardiovascular) exercises for no more than 60 minutes per session, with a combined weekly total not exceeding 200 minutes. Good examples of aerobic exercise include jogging, walking, skipping (with a jump rope) and cycling.

Weight-lifting

As a general rule, always limit weight training to no less than three times per week. During each session, focus on one specific muscle group, as this increases the effectiveness of the workout and reduces the chances of injury.

Never exercise the same muscle groups on consecutive days, as your muscles need the opportunity to recover in between sessions. Training is ineffective if muscles are sore or fatigued, and the chances of contracting an injury are substantially multiplied.

Stretching

Often the most underappreciated form of exercise, stretching is not to be skipped. The excuse of not having the time is not acceptable here, as the consequences of not stretching before and after exercises can be dire.

Although stretching can be done daily, once again it is advisable to limit it to three times a week in order to reap the maximum benefits. The best way to stretch as a form of exercise is after the body is warmed up, in other terms, after a workout. At this time, complete 5 to 10 stretches that target the main muscle groups (especially the ones you have just exercised). It is important to hold each stretch for 10 to 30 seconds in order to get the best results.

When to consult with a doctor first

In many cases, it is wise to see a doctor before commencing any exercise routine. Below is a list of definite pointers to see the doc, but the list is not exhaustive. If you think you should get medical advice for any reason first, trust your instincts and do so.

Consult with your doctor first if:

- You are 45 years old or older

- Physical activity causes pain, especially in your chest area

- You have a history of fainting or dizziness

- Moderate physical activity leaves you breathless

- You are known to have a higher risk of heart disease

- You have heart problems or think you may have heart disease

- You are pregnant. If you are not sure, find out first!

Additional things to remember

If you don't already exercise, start slow. A little exercise is better than no exercise! Commit to doing a little, and gradually build on that.

Aim for an average of 30 minutes of physical activity per day. This can be anything from lifting weights or running, to housework and active chores, to taking a stroll around the block with your dogs. As long as you are moving, it counts!

See everyday activities as new opportunities to be more active. Try parking your car a little farther away and walking the extra distance. If you have a desk job, look up exercises you can do while sitting down. Be sure to take regular breaks away from your desk. Even in small intervals, breaks are hugely beneficial.

If you take public transport, try standing on the bus or train instead of sitting. Take the stairs instead of the lift. Every activity allows for a little more activity.

The best, healthiest and most effective way to lose weight is to combine a healthy diet with exercise. It is the true proven winner and remains effective for almost everyone.

Remember that you cannot out-train a bad diet! They go hand in hand, with diet always trumping exercise.

CITATIONS IN THIS CHAPTER:

(Armand Tecco, 2017)

(Better Health Channel, 2017)

Conclusion

The enormous amounts of confusion abundant in modern-day life are largely unfounded and entirely unnecessary.

The principles behind weight-loss remain the same for everyone, regardless of demographic.

When it comes to proper nutrition, real food always wins. Your body processes it differently to commercially produced foods, and nourishes the body in the way nature intended.

Plant-based diets are generally good ones to follow, as they are based on a naturally-occurring food source that are rich in vitamins and minerals.

Although these meals do require more preparation time, more cooking time and more planning time, the results and better health are far from it. It is senseless to try save 10 minutes on meal preparation and lose 10 years off your life as a result of continued poor food choices.

Any meat dish can be made into a vegetarian or vegan dish – equally delicious and doubly nutritious!

There is no rule that says you cannot eat your favorite foods from time to time, although moderation is key. You may find that with time, your tastes and food preferences change, and you may not like the same unhealthy options that you once did. Furthermore, you will discover more and more ways to make you existing dishes even healthier.

You have the power to change right now. It may be slow and it may be hard, but the rewards are more than worth it. You will feel better and live longer, with the added benefit of enjoying looking in the mirror!

Remember that health and weight loss is not a mystery – it's a science. Old habits die hard, which means that a mental shift is necessary when make a large-scale health and lifestyle change.

Health and weight loss should not be a struggle. The truth is that it's not rocket science – just science!

If you liked this book, please leave a review. It would help me greatly and I would really appreciate it. Thank you for reading.

References

A Calorie Counter. (2017). What is Saturated Fat & Trans Fats? The Unhealthy, Bad Fats. Retrieved from ACalorieCounter.com: http://www.acaloriecounter.com/diet/saturated-fat-trans-fat/

Armand Tecco, M. (2017). Why is Exercise Important? | Health Discovery. Retrieved from HealthDiscovery.Net: http://www.healthdiscovery.net/articles/exercise_importa.htm

Atkins.com. (2017). Recipes | Atkins Low Carb Diet. Retrieved from sa.Atkins.com: https://sa.atkins.com/get-inspired/recipes/

BBC News. (2015, October 26). What is Processed Meat? - BBC News. Retrieved from BBC.com: http://www.bbc.com/news/health-34620617

Better Health Channel. (2017). Physical Activity - It's Important - Better Health Channel. Retrieved from BetterHealth.Vic.Gov.Au:

https://www.betterhealth.vic.gov.au/health/healthy living/physical-activity-its-important

Clear, J. (2017). The Beginner's Guide to Intermittent Fasting. Retrieved from JamesClear.com: https://jamesclear.com/the-beginners-guide-to-intermittent-fasting

Dr. Andreas Eenfeldt, M. (2017, October). A keto diet for beginners - Diet Doctor. Retrieved from DietDoctor.Com: https://www.dietdoctor.com/low-carb/keto

Gluten-Free Living. (2017, May 10). The Basic Gluten-Free Diet - Gluten-Free Living Magazine. Retrieved from GlutenFreeLiving.com: https://www.glutenfreeliving.com/gluten-free-foods/diet/basic-diet/

Health Line. (2017). The Vegan Diet - A complete guide for beginners. Retrieved from HealthLine.com: https://www.healthline.com/nutrition/vegan-diet-guide

Kamb, S. (2010). The Beginner's Guide to the Paleo Diet | NerdFitness. Retrieved from NerdFitness.com:

https://www.nerdfitness.com/blog/the-beginners-guide-to-the-paleo-diet/

Levin, H. (2017). Zero-Calorie Foods List – 21 Fruits & Vegetables to Lose Weight. Retrieved from MoneyCrashers.com: https://www.moneycrashers.com/zero-calorie-foods-list/

Mark Hyman, M. (2016). 5 Reasons Most Diets Fail (And How to Suceed) - Dr. Mark Hyman. Retrieved from DrHyman.com: http://drhyman.com/blog/2014/05/26/5-reasons-diets-fail-succeed/

Mayo Clinic. (2015, April 11). Counting Calories: Get Back to Weight-loss Basics. Retrieved from MayoClinic.org: https://www.mayoclinic.org/healthy-lifestyle/weight-loss/in-depth/calories/art-20048065

Mccaffrey, K. (2012, September 14). How to calculate how much water you should drink a day - Slender Kitchen. Retrieved from www.slenderkitchen.com: https://www.slenderkitchen.com/article/how-to-calculate-how-much-water-you-should-drink-a-day

Men's Fitness. (2017). The Calorie Calculator - How Many
Calories Do You Need? Retrieved from
MensFitness.com:
http://www.mensfitness.com/nutrition/what-to-
eat/the-calorie-calculator-how-many-calories-do-you-
need

NHS Choices. (2016, August 19). Understanding Calories -
Live Well - NHS Choices. Retrieved from NHS.uk:
https://www.nhs.uk/Livewell/loseweight/Pages/u
nderstanding-calories.aspx

Shaw, G. (2017). How Much Water Do You Need? Can You
Drink Too Much? Retrieved from WebMD.com:
https://www.webmd.com/diet/features/water-for-
weight-loss-diet#1

SkillsYouNeed.com. (2017). What is Fat? Good Fats and Bad
Fats | SkillsYouNeed. Retrieved from
SkillsYouNeed.com:
https://www.skillsyouneed.com/ps/fat.html

Slazay, J. (2015, December 10). What is Protein? Retrieved
from LiveScience.com:
https://www.livescience.com/53044-protein.html

Sparacino, A. (2013, July 21). 11 Surprising Health Benefits of Sleep - Health. Retrieved from www.health.com: www.health.com/health/gallery/0,,20459221,00.html

Szalay, J. (2017, July 14). What Are Carbohydrates? Retrieved from LiveScience.com: https://www.livescience.com/51976-carbohydrates.html

The Vegetarian Society. (2016, October). Vegetarian Society - What is a Vegetarian? Retrieved from VegSoc.org: https://www.vegsoc.org/definition

University of Illinois Extension. (2014, June). The Starch and Starchy Vegetables Group | Your Guide to Diet and Diabetes | U of I Extension. Retrieved from Extention.Illinois.edu: http://extension.illinois.edu/diabetes2/subsection.cfm?SubSectionID=19

Weight Watchers UK. (2017). How It Works | Weight Watchers UK. Retrieved from WeightWatchers.com.uk: https://www.weightwatchers.com/uk/how-it-works

Wikipedia. (2017, October 14). Atkins Diet - Wikipedia. Retrieved from en.Wikipedia.org: https://en.wikipedia.org/wiki/Atkins_diet

Wikipedia.org. (2017, October 14). Atkins Diet - Wikipedia. Retrieved from en.Wikipedia.org: https://en.wikipedia.org/wiki/Atkins_diet

Wikipedia.org. (2017, October 19). Ketogenic Diet - Wikipedia. Retrieved from en.Wikipedia.com: https://en.wikipedia.org/wiki/Ketogenic_diet

Wikipedia.org. (2017, October 22). Paleolithic Diet - Wikipedia. Retrieved from en.Wikipedia.org: https://en.wikipedia.org/wiki/Paleolithic_diet

Winston, D. C. (2017). List of Refined Carbs | Healthy Living | Sf Gate. Retrieved from HealthyLiving.sfgate.com: http://healthyeating.sfgate.com/list-refined-carbs-7260.html